Disclaimer The information provided in this eBook is for general informational purposes only. While the author and publisher have made every effort to ensure the accuracy and completeness of the information contained in this book, they assume no responsibility for errors, omissions, or contrary interpretations of the subject matter herein. The information is provided on an "as is" basis, and the author and publisher shall have neither liability nor responsibility to any person or entity with respect to any loss or damages arising from the information contained in this eBook.

Table Of Contents

Chapter 1: Introduction to Home Workout Hustle

The Benefits of Home Workouts for Weight Loss, Muscle Building, and Strength Training and more for Beginners

Home workouts can be a game-changer for busy individuals who want to prioritize their health and fitness. Not only are they convenient and time-saving, but weight loss is one of the most significant benefits of home workouts for beginners. They also offer many benefits for beginners looking to kickstart their fitness journey. This subchapter will explore the various advantages of home workouts, including weight loss, muscle building, and strength training.

Engaging in regular exercise routines from home can effectively burn calories and shed excess pounds. Whether you prefer high-intensity interval training (HIIT), circuit training, or cardio workouts, plenty of options can help you achieve your weight-loss goals. Additionally, incorporating accessories such as dumbbells, resistance bands, or a treadmill can enhance the effectiveness of your workouts and accelerate your progress.

In addition to weight loss, home workouts are also excellent for building muscle and toning your body. Strength training exercises, such as squats, lunges, push-ups, and planks, can help you target specific muscle groups and improve your overall strength and endurance. By gradually increasing the intensity of your workouts and challenging your muscles, you can achieve noticeable gains in muscle mass and definition over time. With the proper guidance and consistency, you can transform your physique and achieve the desired results without ever setting foot in a gym.

Moreover, strength training is essential to any fitness routine, as it helps improve your overall health and functional fitness. Regularly engaging in resistance training exercises can increase bone density, boost metabolism, and enhance balance and coordination. These benefits are significant for beginners looking to improve their physical fitness and prevent age-related muscle loss. With the proper home workout routines and accessories, you can effectively strengthen your muscles and joints and maintain a healthy and active lifestyle for years.

In conclusion, home workouts offer many benefits for beginners who prioritize their health and fitness journey. Whether your goal is to lose weight, build muscle, or improve your strength and endurance, plenty of home workout routines can help you achieve your desired results. By incorporating accessories such as dumbbells, resistance bands, or a treadmill into your workouts, you can enhance the effectiveness of your exercises and maximize your progress. With dedication, consistency, and the proper guidance, you can transform your body and elevate your fitness level from the comfort of your home. https://www.nerdfitness.com/blog/the-7-best-at-home-workout-routines-the-ultimate-guide-for-training-without-a-gym/

https://greatist.com/fitness/at-home-workouts-for-beginners

https://www.verywellfit.com/easy-workouts-for-beginners-3496020

Overcoming Common Excuses

Overcoming common excuses is essential for busy individuals who are looking to make their health a priority. It's easy to come up with reasons why you can't fit exercise into your schedule, but with the right mindset and tools, you can overcome these obstacles. One common excuse is lack of time, but with the proper home workout routine, you can get a quick and effective workout quickly. By prioritizing your health, you can start seeing improvements in your overall well-being.

Another common excuse is a lack of equipment, but many accessories can be helpful in a home workout routine. Dumbbells, resistance bands, a treadmill, and a yoga mat are just a few examples of equipment that can help you get a great workout in the comfort of your home. These accessories are affordable and easy to use, making them perfect for busy individuals who want to prioritize their health and are short on time.

It's also common to use a lack of motivation as an excuse for not working out. However, by finding a routine you enjoy and setting achievable goals, you can stay motivated and committed to your fitness journey. Whether following a specific workout plan or joining a virtual fitness class, there are many ways to stay motivated and overcome this common excuse.

Another common excuse is feeling too tired to exercise after a long day at work. However, regular exercise can increase energy levels and improve overall mood. Making exercise a regular part of your routine makes you feel more energized and motivated to continue working towards your health and fitness goals.

In conclusion, overcoming common excuses is essential for busy individuals who want to prioritize their health. By finding a home workout routine that works for you, investing in valuable accessories, staying motivated, and making exercise a regular part of your routine, you can overcome these obstacles and improve your overall well-being. With the right mindset and tools, you can achieve your health and fitness goals, even with a busy schedule.

https://theheartfoundation.org/2018/06/01/the-top-10-excuses-for-not-exercising-and-solutions/

https://fitonapp.com/fitness/exercise-excuses/

Essential Accessories for Home Workouts

Having the right accessories on hand is essential to maximizing the effectiveness of your home workout routines. Whether short on time or space, having the proper equipment can make all the difference in achieving your fitness goals. From dumbbells to resistance bands, there are a variety of accessories that can help take your home workouts to the next level.

A set of dumbbells is one of the most versatile and essential accessories for home workouts. Dumbbells allow you to target specific muscle groups and vary the intensity of your exercises. Whether you're looking to build strength, increase endurance, or tone your muscles, having a set of dumbbells in various weights can help you achieve your fitness goals.

Another must-have accessory for home workouts is a treadmill. While running outdoors is a great way to get your cardio in, having a treadmill at home can provide a convenient and weather-proof option for those days you can't go outside. With a treadmill, you can easily fit in a quick run or walk without worrying about traffic, weather, or time constraints.

Resistance bands are another essential accessory for home workouts. These versatile bands can target specific muscle groups, increase flexibility, and add resistance to your exercises. Whether you want to tone your arms, strengthen your legs, or improve your balance, resistance bands can help you achieve your fitness goals without taking up much space.

A stability ball is an excellent accessory for those looking to add variety to their home workout routines. Stability balls can improve balance, core strength, and flexibility. They can also modify traditional exercises, making them more challenging and engaging. A stability ball can help take your workouts to the next level, whether you're doing crunches, planks, or squats.

In conclusion, having the right accessories for your home workouts can significantly improve the effectiveness and enjoyment of your fitness routine.

Whether you invest in dumbbells, a treadmill, resistance bands, or a stability ball, having the right equipment can help you achieve your fitness goals in the comfort of your home. So don't let a busy schedule stop prioritizing your health; invest in the essential accessories for home workouts and start hustling towards a healthier you today. https://www.goodhousekeeping.com/health-products/g26951456/best-home-gym-equipment/

https://barbend.com/best-home-gym-equipment/

Chapter 2: Setting Up Your Home Workout Space

Choosing the Right Space

Choosing a suitable space for your home workout routine is crucial to staying consistent and motivated in your fitness journey. When selecting a space, consider size, lighting, and ventilation. A space that is too small can limit your range of motion and make it difficult to perform specific exercises. On the other hand, a too-large space may feel overwhelming and lack the cozy atmosphere needed for a successful workout.

When it comes to lighting, natural light is always the best option, as it can help boost your mood and energy levels. Opt for bright artificial lighting that mimics natural sunlight if natural light is unavailable. Additionally, ensure your workout space is well-ventilated to prevent overheating and ensure proper airflow during your workouts. Proper ventilation can also help reduce the buildup of sweat and odors, creating a more pleasant environment for your workouts.

Consider the layout of your workout space and how it can accommodate the equipment you will be using. If you plan on incorporating accessories such as dumbbells, resistance bands, or a treadmill, ensure enough space to move around comfortably and safely. Storage solutions are also essential to keep your equipment organized and easily accessible. This can help streamline your workouts and prevent any unnecessary interruptions due to clutter.

In addition to the physical aspects of your workout space, consider the atmosphere and ambiance you want to create. Choose a space that feels inviting and motivating, whether that means adding plants, motivational quotes, or your favorite workout playlist. Creating a space that you enjoy being in can help you look forward to your workouts and stay committed to your fitness goals. Remember, your workout space reflects your dedication to your health and well-being, so choose wisely.

A suitable workout space inspires and energizes you to push yourself to new limits. Take the time to assess your needs and preferences when selecting a space for your home workouts. By creating a comfortable, well-equipped, and motivating space, you can set yourself up for success in achieving your fitness goals. Making your health a priority, even amid a busy schedule, is possible with a suitable space and mindset.

Organizing Your Equipment

The right equipment is essential for maximizing your results when working out at home. Organizing your equipment is critical to ensuring your home workout space is efficient and clutter-free. This subchapter will discuss the importance of arranging your equipment and provide tips on how to do so effectively.

First and foremost, taking stock of your equipment and assessing what you need for your workouts is essential. For busy individuals, having a few critical pieces of equipment that can be used for multiple exercises is ideal. Dumbbells, resistance bands, a stability ball, and a yoga mat are versatile accessories that can be used for a variety of exercises and can easily be stored in a small space.

Once you have identified the equipment you need, it is time to consider how to store and organize it in your home workout space. Investing in storage solutions such as shelves, bins, or a workout bench with built-in storage can help keep your equipment organized and easily accessible. Consider designating specific areas for different types of equipment to make it easier to find what you need during your workouts.

Another essential aspect of organizing your equipment is keeping it in good condition. Regularly cleaning and maintaining your equipment will prolong its lifespan and ensure its safety. Make sure to wipe down your equipment after each use, store it in a dry and clean area, and check for any signs of wear and tear that may require repairs or replacement.

In conclusion, organizing your equipment is crucial for creating a functional and efficient home workout space. By taking stock of your equipment, investing in storage solutions, and maintaining your equipment correctly, you can ensure that your home workouts are effective and enjoyable. Remember, a well-organized workout space can help you stay motivated and committed to your fitness goals, even when you are short on time. https://trugrit-fitness.com/blogs/news/home-gym-storage

https://trugrit-fitness.com/blogs/news/home-gym-storage

Creating a Motivating Atmosphere

Creating a motivating atmosphere is essential for sticking to your home workout routine, especially for busy individuals trying to prioritize their health despite their hectic schedules. One critical element of a motivating atmosphere is having the right accessories. Investing in equipment such as dumbbells, resistance bands, a yoga mat, or even a treadmill can help you stay motivated and make your workouts more effective. Creating a motivating and effective home workout atmosphere is essential for staying consistent and achieving your fitness goals. Here are some tips to help you set up an inspiring workout space:

1. **Designate a dedicated living room corner area:**

   - Choose a specific area in your home where you'll do your workouts. It could be a spare room, a corner of your living room, or even your garage.
   - Having a designated space helps mentally prepare you for exercise.

2. **Clear the clutter:**

o   Remove any unnecessary items from your workout area. A clutter-free space allows you to focus better.

o   Consider using storage bins or shelves to keep your workout accessories organized.

3. **Lighting Matters**:

o   Natural light is ideal, but if that's not possible, install bright LED lights.

o   Good lighting can boost your mood and make the space more inviting.

4. **Mirrors for Form Check**:

o   Hang a full-length mirror or place smaller mirrors strategically.

o   Mirrors create a sense of space and allow you to check your form during exercises.

5. **Motivational Decor**:

o   Add motivational quotes, posters, or pictures of fitness role models.

o   Personalize the space to make it feel inspiring and uplifting.

6. **Sound System**:

o   Set up a small speaker or Bluetooth device for music or workout videos.

o   Music can energize you during workouts.

1. **Flooring**:

o   Invest in a good-quality yoga mat or exercise mat. This provides cushioning and prevents slipping during exercises.

o   Consider adding foam tiles or interlocking rubber mats if you have a hard floor.

2. **Plants and greenery**:

- o Indoor plants improve air quality and add a refreshing touch to your workout area.
   - o Choose low-maintenance plants that thrive indoors.
3. **Organize Your Equipment**:

   - o Use hooks, shelves, or wall-mounted racks to store your resistance bands, dumbbells, and other accessories.
   - o Keep frequently used items within easy reach.
4. **Personalize Your Playlist**:

   Create a workout playlist with your favorite tunes. Music can boost your motivation and make workouts more enjoyable.

5. **Comfortable Attire**:

   - o Wear comfortable workout clothes that make you feel good.
   - o Having a designated workout outfit can mentally prepare you for exercise.
6. **Set the mood**:

   - o Consider using scented candles or essential oils to create a pleasant atmosphere.
   - o Find scents that relax or energize you, depending on the type of workout.

Remember, your home workout atmosphere should reflect your personality and preferences. Make it a space where you look forward to sweating it out and achieving your fitness goals!

A dedicated workout space can also significantly affect your motivation to exercise. Whether it's a corner of your living room, a spare bedroom, or even a cleared-out area in your garage, having a designated space for your workouts can help you get into the right mindset and make it easier to stay on track with your fitness goals. Ensure your workout space is clean, clutter-free, and well-lit to help create a positive and motivating environment.

Another way to create a motivating atmosphere for your home workouts is by setting specific goals for yourself. Whether you're aiming to increase your strength, improve your endurance, or simply try to be consistent with your workouts, having clear goals in mind can help keep you focused and motivated. Write down your goals and keep them somewhere visible in your workout space as a constant reminder of what you're working towards.

Listening to upbeat music or podcasts can also help create a motivating atmosphere for your home workouts. Create a playlist of your favorite songs that get you pumped up and ready to exercise, or listen to motivational podcasts that inspire you to keep pushing yourself. Having something to listen to while you work out can help keep you energized and motivated throughout your workout.

Finally, surrounding yourself with positive reinforcement can help create a motivating atmosphere for your home workouts. Whether through virtual workout buddies, online fitness communities, or simply sharing your progress with friends and family, having a support system can help keep you accountable and motivated to stick to your routine. Celebrate your successes, no matter how small, and use them as motivation to keep pushing yourself towards your fitness goals.

Chapter 3: The Basics of Home Workouts

Understanding Different Types of Exercises

To make the most of your home workouts, it is essential to understand the different types of exercises you can incorporate into your routine. By diversifying your exercises, you can target different muscle groups and prevent boredom from setting in. In this subchapter, we will explore the various types of exercises that you can incorporate into your home workout routine.

Strength training exercises are essential for building muscle and increasing strength. These exercises typically involve using resistance, such as dumbbells or resistance bands, to work against the force of gravity. Examples of strength-training exercises include squats, lunges, push-ups, and bicep curls. Incorporating these exercises into your routine can build lean muscle mass and boost metabolism. https://www.healthline.com/health/exercise-fitness/strength-training-at-home

Cardiovascular exercises are essential for improving heart health and burning calories. They typically elevate your heart rate and increase your breathing rate. Examples of cardiovascular exercises include running, cycling, jumping jacks, and high knees. By incorporating cardiovascular exercises into your routine, you can improve your endurance and stamina, burn fat, and lose weight. https://www.healthline.com/health/cardio-exercises-at-home

Flexibility exercises are essential for improving the range of motion and preventing injuries. They typically involve stretching and lengthening the muscles. Examples of flexibility exercises include yoga, Pilates, and static stretching. Incorporating flexibility exercises into your routine can improve overall mobility and reduce the risk of injury during workouts.

Improving flexibility at home is reasonably achievable with the right exercises. Here are some effective flexibility exercises that you can incorporate into your routine:

1. **Neck and Shoulder Stretches**:

Tilt your head to one side, bringing your ear towards the shoulder, until you feel a stretch.

- Roll your shoulders slowly in a circular motion to relieve tension.

2. **Cat-Cow Stretch**:

- On all fours, alternate between arching your back towards the ceiling (Cat) and dipping it towards the floor (Cow).

- This exercise is excellent for spinal flexibility and relieving back tension.

3. **Seated Forward Bend**:

Sit with your legs extended in front of you.

- Reach forward towards your toes, keeping your back straight.

- Hold the stretch to feel a deep stretch in your hamstrings and lower back.

4. **Butterfly Stretch**:

- Sit with the soles of your feet together and your knees out to the sides.

-Press your knees with your elbows or hands to stretch your inner thighs.

5. **Tricep Stretch**:

- Raise one arm overhead, then bend the elbow so your hand reaches the opposite shoulder blade.

- Use the other hand to gently press on the bent elbow for a deeper stretch.

6. **Cobra Pose**:

- Lie on your stomach with your hands under your shoulders.

- Gently lift your chest off the ground, extending through the spine.

- This stretch is excellent for the flexibility of the lower back and abdominal muscles.

7. **Child's Pose**:

- From a kneeling position, sit back on your heels and stretch your arms forward on the floor.

- Lower your forehead to the ground and relax into the stretch.

8. **Standing Quadriceps Stretch**:

- Stand on one leg, grab the other foot with your hand, and pull it towards your glutes.

- Keep your knees close together and maintain balance.

9. **Lunging Hip Flexor Stretch**:

- Step one foot forward into a lunge position.

- Lower your back knee to the ground and lean forward to stretch the hip flexors of the back leg.

10. **Standing Calf Stretch**:

- Place your hands on a wall and extend one leg back, keeping the heel on the ground.

- Lean forward with the other leg bent, feeling the stretch in the calf of the extended leg.

Remember to breathe deeply and hold each stretch for 15 to 30 seconds. Consistency is key, so try to incorporate these stretches into your daily routine for the best results. Happy stretching!

The 25 Best Beginner Stretches for Flexibility—Greatest.
https://greatist.com/fitness/beginner-stretches-for-flexibility.

How to Improve Flexibility (in 30 Days) | Nerd Fitness.
https://www.nerdfitness.com/blog/the-3-best-flexibility-exercises-the-ultimate-guide-for-improving-flexibility-in-30-days/.

How to Be More Flexible: 30 Tips, Stretches, Exercises, and More.
https://www.healthline.com/health/fitness-exercise/how-to-be-more-flexible.

15-Minute Beginner Stretch Flexibility Routine! (FOLLOW ALONG).
https://www.youtube.com/watch?v=L_xrDAtykMI.

10-MIN STRETCHING EXERCISES FOR STIFF MUSCLES AT HOME (Relaxation & Flexibility) | No Equipment.
https://www.youtube.com/watch?v=YfCK3uOz1r4.

25-MIN STRETCH & CORE: Full Body Recovery (Mobility, Flexibility Workout at Home), no equipment.
https://www.youtube.com/watch?v=R0eqxnSyRkM.

Four types of exercise can improve your health and physical ability.
https://www.nia.nih.gov/health/exercise-and-physical-activity/four-types-exercise-can-improve-your-health-and-physical.

Balance exercises are essential for improving coordination, stability, and posture. These exercises typically challenge your ability to maintain your center of gravity. Examples of balance exercises include single-leg stands, heel-to-toe walks, and stability ball exercises. Incorporating balance exercises into your routine can improve overall balance and coordination and reduce the risk of falls and injuries.

Functional exercises are essential for improving everyday movements and activities. These exercises typically mimic real-life movements and engage multiple muscle groups at once. Examples of functional exercises include squats with a shoulder press, lunges with a twist, and plank rows. Incorporating functional exercises into your routine can improve your overall strength, stability, and coordination and enhance your performance in daily activities.

Proper Warm-up and Cool-down Techniques

Proper warm-up and cool-down techniques are essential to any successful workout routine, especially for busy individuals looking to prioritize their health. By properly preparing your body for exercise and allowing it to recover safely afterward, you can maximize the benefits of your workouts and reduce the risk of injury.

Before starting any workout, spending at least 5–10 minutes warming up your muscles and increasing your heart rate is essential. This can be done through activities such as jogging in place, jumping jacks, or dynamic stretches. By gradually increasing the intensity of your warm-up, you can help improve blood flow to your muscles and joints, making them more flexible and ready for the workout ahead.

After completing your workout, it is equally important to cool down properly to help your body recover. This can be done by performing static stretches to help lengthen your muscles and reduce soreness. Cooling down can also help lower your heart rate and prevent dizziness or lightheadedness after intense exercise.

In addition to proper warm-up and cool-down techniques, busy health enthusiasts can benefit from incorporating accessories such as dumbbells, resistance bands, or a treadmill into their home workout routines. These tools can help add variety and challenge to your workouts, allowing you to target different muscle groups and make the most of your limited time.

By prioritizing proper warm-up and cool-down techniques and utilizing helpful accessories, busy individuals can ensure they are getting the most out of their home workout routines. Making your health a priority doesn't have to be time-consuming, and by following these simple guidelines, you can stay on track with your fitness goals while still managing your busy schedule.

https://barbend.com/cool-down-exercises/

https://www.mayoclinic.org/healthy-lifestyle/fitness/in-depth/exercise/art-20045517pushing ourselves to the limit with every workout can be tempting

Importance of Rest and Recovery

Rest and recovery are often overlooked aspects of any fitness routine, but they are crucial for achieving optimal results. As busy individuals constantly on the go, it can be tempting to push ourselves to the limit with every workout. However, failing to prioritize rest and recovery can lead to burnout and injury and ultimately hinder our progress toward our health and fitness goals.

Our muscles undergo stress and microtears when we engage in intense physical activity. It is during rest and recovery that our muscles have the opportunity to repair and grow stronger. Without adequate rest, our muscles do not have the chance to recover fully, which can lead to decreased performance and an increased risk of injury. Additionally, rest and recovery play a crucial role in preventing overtraining and mental fatigue, allowing us to maintain motivation and consistency in our workout routines.

Incorporating rest and recovery into our busy schedules can be challenging but essential for our overall health and well-being. By prioritizing sleep, hydration, and proper nutrition, we can support our body's recovery process and ensure we are ready to tackle our next workout with total energy and focus. Additionally, active recovery activities such as yoga, stretching, or low-intensity cardio can help promote blood flow and alleviate muscle soreness.

Rest and recovery become even more critical to your health, and fitness goals become more achievable with in-home workouts, as we may not have access to the same resources and amenities as a traditional gym. Investing in accessories such as foam rollers, resistance bands, and massage balls can aid in our recovery process and help alleviate muscle tension. Additionally, incorporating restorative practices such as meditation and deep breathing exercises can help calm the mind and promote relaxation, further enhancing our body's ability to recover.

In conclusion, rest and recovery are vital components of any fitness routine, especially for busy individuals constantly juggling multiple responsibilities. By prioritizing rest, proper nutrition, and active recovery activities, we can support our body's repair process and ensure that we are able to perform at our best in each workout. Remember, it is not just about the intensity of our workouts but also about how well we take care of our bodies in between. Make rest and recovery a priority and watch as your health and fitness goals become more achievable than ever before.

https://www.canr.msu.edu/news/the_importance_of_rest_and_recovery_for_at hletes https://www.verywellfit.com/the-benefits-of-rest-and-recovery-after-exercise-3120575

Chapter 4: Top 10 Home Workout Routines and what that would look like for a home workout with sets and reps with accessories

Full-body HIIT Workout

This subchapter will explore the benefits of a full-body high-intensity interval training (HIIT) workout for busy individuals looking to prioritize their health and fitness. HIIT workouts are known for their efficiency in burning calories and increasing cardiovascular endurance quickly, making them ideal for those with hectic schedules. By incorporating a variety of exercises that target multiple muscle groups simultaneously, a full-body HIIT workout can help you maximize your time and see results quickly.

To start your full-body HIIT workout, you will need minimal equipment such as dumbbells, resistance bands, a jump rope, or a treadmill. These accessories can help you add resistance and intensity to your exercises, allowing you to challenge yourself and push your limits. Utilizing these tools can help you create a well-rounded workout routine that engages all major muscle groups and enables you to effectively burn calories and shed excess pounds by exercising regularly at home to achieve a balanced physique.

One key component of a full-body HIIT workout is interval training. This involves alternating between periods of high-intensity exercise and short rest periods. By pushing yourself to work at maximum effort during the high-intensity intervals, you can elevate your heart rate and boost your metabolism, leading to increased calorie burn and improved cardiovascular health. The short rest periods allow you to recover and catch your breath before diving back into the next set, keeping the intensity high throughout the workout.

Some sample exercises included in a full-body HIIT workout are burpees, mountain climbers, squats, lunges, push-ups, and plank variations. These exercises simultaneously engage multiple muscle groups, providing a comprehensive workout that targets the upper body, lower body, and core. By performing these exercises in quick succession with minimal rest in between, you can keep your heart rate up and maximize calorie burn. Additionally, incorporating a mix of strength training and cardio exercises helps you build muscle, increase endurance, and improve overall fitness levels.

In conclusion, a full-body HIIT workout is a time-efficient and effective way for busy individuals to prioritize their health and fitness goals. You can create a challenging and dynamic workout routine that yields results by utilizing minimal equipment and performing various exercises targeting multiple muscle groups. Whether you're a beginner or a seasoned fitness enthusiast, incorporating HIIT workouts into your routine can help you stay on track with your health and wellness journey, even when time is limited.
https://www.verywellfit.com/basic-full-body-workout-you-can-do-at-home-1231515

Cardio Blast Circuit

The Cardio Blast Circuit is one of the most effective routines in the Home Workout Hustle book, designed specifically for busy individuals who want to prioritize their health. This intense circuit combines high-intensity cardio exercises with strength training to provide a full-body workout in a short amount of time. You can quickly complete this challenging routine in your home with the right accessories, such as dumbbells, a treadmill, and resistance bands.

To begin the cardio blast circuit, start with a quick warm-up to prepare your muscles for the intense workout. This can include jumping jacks, high knees, and arm circles to raise your heart rate and increase blood flow to your muscles. Once warmed up, move on to the first set of exercises, which may include burpees, mountain climbers, and squat jumps, to engage multiple muscle groups and increase cardiovascular endurance.

As you progress through the circuit, push yourself to your limits while maintaining proper form to prevent injury. Use dumbbells for lunges, bicep curls, and shoulder presses to add resistance and challenge your muscles even further. The treadmill can be incorporated for sprinting or incline walking intervals to elevate your heart rate and burn more calories.

In between each set of exercises, take short breaks to catch your breath and hydrate with water to stay energized throughout the circuit. Listen to your body and modify exercises to accommodate your fitness level. By the end of the Cardio Blast Circuit, you will have completed a high-intensity workout that targets all major muscle groups and improves your cardiovascular health.

Incorporating the Cardio Blast Circuit into your weekly routine will help you stay fit and healthy and save time by eliminating the need to commute to the gym. With the right accessories and dedication, you can achieve your fitness goals from the comfort of your own home. So, lace up your sneakers, grab your dumbbells, and get ready to sweat with the Cardio Blast Circuit!

Upper Body Strength Training

Upper body strength training is essential to any fitness routine, as it helps build muscle mass, increase metabolism, and improve overall strength and endurance. For busy individuals looking to prioritize their health and fitness goals, incorporating upper-body strength training exercises into their workout routine can be a highly effective way to achieve their desired results. This subchapter will explore some of the top exercises and routines that can be done at home with minimal equipment, such as dumbbells, resistance bands, or just body weight.

One of the most effective upper-body strength training exercises is the push-up. Push-ups work the muscles in the chest, shoulders, and triceps and can be modified to accommodate different fitness levels. For beginners, modified push-ups can be done on the knees, while more advanced individuals can perform traditional push-ups on their toes. Push-ups can be done in sets of 10–15 repetitions, with 3–4 sets for a complete upper-body workout.

Another excellent exercise for building upper-body strength is the dumbbell shoulder press. This exercise targets the shoulders, triceps, and upper back muscles and can be done with either a pair of dumbbells or a single dumbbell held in both hands. To perform a dumbbell shoulder press, sit or stand with a dumbbell in each hand, palms facing forward. Press the dumbbells overhead until your arms are fully extended, then lower them back down to shoulder level. Aim for 3–4 sets of 10–12 repetitions for a challenging upper-body workout.

In addition to push-ups and dumbbell shoulder presses, incorporating exercises like bicep curls, tricep dips, and chest flyes can help target specific muscles in the upper body and provide a well-rounded strength training routine. Individuals can effectively challenge their muscles and progress toward their fitness goals by combining different exercises and varying the number of sets and repetitions. It is essential to listen to your body and adjust the intensity of your workouts as needed to prevent injury and promote recovery.

For busy individuals who may not have access to a full range of gym equipment, there are still plenty of options for practical upper-body strength training at home. Resistance bands can add variety and resistance to exercises like rows, pull-a-parts, and chest presses. Bodyweight exercises like planks, mountain climbers, and tricep dips can also be done with minimal equipment and provide a challenging workout for the upper body. By incorporating these exercises into a regular workout routine, busy individuals can prioritize their health and see actual results in their strength and fitness levels.

https://www.verywellfit.com/beginner-upper-body-workout-get-started-on-your-upper-body-1231520

https://www.livestrong.com/article/13721708-upper-body-at-home-workout-beginners/

Lower Body Booty Burn

In the world of fitness, the quest for a toned and sculpted lower body is a common goal for many individuals. However, finding the time to hit the gym and focus on targeted exercises can be challenging, especially for busy individuals who are constantly on the go. That's where the "Lower Body Booty Burn" routine comes in—a high-intensity workout designed to target and strengthen the muscles of the lower body, all from the comfort of your own home.

To start with the Lower Body Booty, Burn routine, you only need a set of dumbbells and a yoga mat. These simple accessories can help enhance the workout's effectiveness by adding resistance and stability to your movements. Dumbbells can be used for squats, lunges, and deadlifts, while a yoga mat can provide a comfortable surface for floor exercises like glute bridges and leg lifts.

The Lower Body Booty Burn routine consists of compound exercises that target multiple muscle groups at once, helping to increase strength and build lean muscle mass in the lower body. This helps sculpt and tone your legs, glutes, and thighs, boosts your metabolism, and burns calories long after the workout. This routine is designed to maximize your time and effort for maximum results by incorporating strength training and cardio exercises.

One key benefit of the Lower Body Booty Burn routine is its versatility and adaptability to different fitness levels. Whether you're a beginner looking to build strength or an experienced athlete seeking a new challenge, this workout can be modified to suit your needs and goals. By adjusting each exercise's weight, reps, and intensity, you can tailor the routine to your fitness level and progress at your own pace.

In conclusion, the Lower Body Booty Burn routine is a quick and effective workout that can help busy individuals prioritize their health and fitness goals. You can achieve a challenging and rewarding workout without leaving your home by incorporating targeted lower-body exercises and simple accessories like dumbbells and a yoga mat. So why wait? Lace up your sneakers, grab your dumbbells, and get ready to feel the burn with this dynamic lower-body routine.

Core Crusher Abs Routine

In this subchapter, we will focus on a Core Crusher Abs Routine that is perfect for busy individuals who want to prioritize their health and fitness. This routine is designed to target your core muscles and help you achieve a strong and toned midsection. By incorporating this routine into your regular workout schedule, you can improve your overall strength and stability and enhance your athletic performance.

To perform this Core Crusher Abs Routine, you will need minimal accessories, such as a yoga mat and a set of dumbbells. These items will help you enhance the effectiveness of the exercises and provide added resistance for a more challenging workout. Additionally, if you have access to a treadmill or other cardio equipment, you can further incorporate some high-intensity intervals to boost your calorie burn and cardiovascular fitness.

The Core Crusher Abs Routine consists of a series of exercises that target all areas of the core, including the upper and lower abs, obliques, and lower back muscles. Some of the critical exercises included in this routine are planks, Russian twists, leg raises, and bicycle crunches. These exercises are designed to engage multiple muscle groups simultaneously, helping you achieve a more efficient and effective workout in less time.

Regularly following this Core Crusher Abs Routine can strengthen your core muscles, improve your posture, and reduce your risk of injury during physical activities. A strong core can help you perform everyday tasks more efficiently and with less strain on your body. So, this routine is perfect for you, whether you are a busy professional, a parent juggling multiple responsibilities, or someone who simply wants to prioritize their health.

In conclusion, the Core Crusher Abs Routine is an excellent addition to any home workout routine for busy individuals looking to improve their fitness and health. By dedicating just a few minutes each day to this routine, you can see significant improvements in your core strength and stability. So, grab your accessories, clear some space in your living room, and get ready to crush your core with this practical and efficient workout routine.

https://www.facebook.com/hardcoreainsley/videos/core-crusher-add-this-killer-ab-circuit-to-the-end-of-your-workouts-this-weekv-u/983806319387291/

Dumbbell Power Workout

The dumbbell power workout is a highly effective routine for busy individuals who want to prioritize their health and fitness. This workout is designed to build strength and muscle mass using dumbbells, making it a convenient option for those who may not have access to a complete gym setup. By incorporating dumbbells into your routine, you can target multiple muscle groups and challenge your body in new ways.

To begin the dumbbell power workout, start with a warm-up to prepare your muscles for the exercises. This can include dynamic stretches, light cardio, or bodyweight exercises. Once you are warmed up, choose a pair of challenging but manageable dumbbells for the exercises you will be performing. Maintaining proper form throughout the workout is essential to prevent injury and maximize results.

The Dumbbell Power Workout consists of exercises targeting different muscle groups, such as squats, lunges, chest presses, rows, and shoulder presses. These exercises are designed to be performed in a circuit format, completing each exercise for a set number of repetitions before moving on to the next. This format helps elevate your heart rate and maximize calorie burn while building strength and muscle.

Incorporating the Dumbbell Power Workout into your routine can help you see results quickly, making it ideal for busy individuals. Committing to this workout a few times a week can improve your strength, muscle tone, and overall fitness level. With just a pair of dumbbells and a small space to work out in, you can easily fit this routine into your busy schedule.

The dumbbell power workout is a versatile and efficient routine that can help busy individuals achieve their fitness goals. By incorporating this workout into your routine, you can improve your strength, muscle mass, and overall health without the need for a full gym setup. Make your health a priority by investing in a pair of dumbbells and committing to this challenging and rewarding workout. https://stronghomegym.com/full-body-dumbbell-workout/

Resistance Band Sculpt

Resistance bands are a versatile and convenient tool for sculpting your body in the comfort of your own home. These bands come in various levels of resistance, making them suitable for individuals of all fitness levels. Incorporating resistance band exercises into your workout routine can help tone and strengthen your muscles, improve flexibility, and increase overall endurance.

One key benefit of resistance band sculpting is its ability to target specific muscle groups precisely. You can effectively work your arms, legs, chest, back, and core by using different resistance levels and adjusting your body positioning. This targeted approach allows you to tailor your workouts to focus on areas that need attention, helping you achieve your fitness goals more efficiently.

In addition to targeting specific muscle groups, resistance band sculpting helps improve overall muscle stability and coordination. The bands' constant tension forces your muscles to work harder throughout each exercise, increasing muscle activation and engagement. This leads to better muscle tone and definition and enhances physical performance in other activities.

Another advantage of resistance band sculpting is the portability and affordability of the equipment. Unlike bulky and expensive gym equipment like dumbbells or treadmills, resistance bands are lightweight, compact, and budget-friendly. This makes them an ideal option for busy individuals who want to stay active and fit without the need for an entire home gym setup. You can easily store and carry resistance bands wherever you go, allowing you to squeeze in a quick workout anytime, anywhere.

Overall, resistance band sculpting is a highly effective and efficient way to improve your fitness level and achieve your health goals. Whether you are a beginner looking to build strength or an experienced athlete wanting to enhance your performance, incorporating resistance bands into your workout routine can help take your workouts to the next level. With a variety of exercises and routines to choose from, you can keep your workouts challenging and engaging while sculpting a leaner, stronger, and healthier body. https://thefitnessphantom.com/the-full-body-resistance-band-workout

Treadmill Interval Training

Treadmill interval training is a highly effective and time-efficient workout routine that can help busy individuals achieve their fitness goals. This type of workout involves alternating between high-intensity running or sprinting and periods of lower-intensity recovery or walking on the treadmill. By incorporating intervals into your treadmill workout, you can burn more calories, improve cardiovascular fitness, and increase overall endurance in a shorter amount of time.

To start a treadmill interval training session, begin with a 5–10-minute warm-up at a moderate pace to prepare your body for the upcoming workout. Once warmed up, increase the speed and incline of the treadmill to a challenging level for 30–60 seconds of high-intensity running or sprinting. After completing the high-intensity interval, reduce the speed and incline to a comfortable level for 60–90 seconds of recovery walking or jogging. Repeat this cycle for 10–20 minutes, depending on your fitness level and goals.

One key benefit of treadmill interval training is its ability to boost metabolism and burn calories long after the workout. The high-intensity intervals create an "afterburn" effect, known as excess post-exercise oxygen consumption (EPOC), which increases the number of calories burned post-workout. This can help busy individuals maximize their time and effort toward achieving weight loss or maintenance goals.

In addition to burning calories and improving cardiovascular fitness, treadmill interval training can help increase overall endurance and stamina. By pushing your body to work at higher intensities during the intervals, you can improve your body's ability to sustain physical activity for longer periods of time. This can be especially beneficial for busy individuals who may have limited time for exercise but still want to see improvements in their fitness levels.

Overall, treadmill interval training is a versatile and effective workout routine that can be easily incorporated into a busy lifestyle. Utilizing the treadmill and incorporating intervals into your workout can maximize your time, burn more calories, and improve your overall fitness. Whether you are a beginner looking to kickstart your fitness journey or a seasoned athlete looking to challenge yourself, treadmill interval training is an excellent option for busy health enthusiasts looking to prioritize their health and well-being.

https://www.runnersblueprint.com/maximize-your-treadmill-time-a-30-minute-hiit-workout-for-beginners/

Yoga Flow for Flexibility

Yoga Flow for Flexibility is a crucial routine for busy individuals who want to prioritize their health and well-being. This routine focuses on improving flexibility, mobility, and overall body awareness through a series of flowing yoga poses. Incorporating this routine into your weekly schedule can increase your range of motion, reduce the risk of injury, and enhance your overall physical performance.

To begin the Yoga Flow for Flexibility routine, start in a comfortable seated position on your mat. Take a few deep breaths to center yourself and focus on the present moment. From there, move into a gentle warm-up sequence that includes cat-cow stretches, spinal twists, and gentle neck stretches. These movements help to loosen up the muscles and prepare your body for the more dynamic poses.

As you progress through the routine, you will move through a series of standing and seated poses that target different areas of the body. Poses such as Downward Facing Dog, Warrior II, and Triangle Pose helps to stretch and strengthen the legs, hips, and core muscles. Other poses, such as Child's Pose and Pigeon Pose, target the lower back, hips, and glutes, helping to release tension and improve overall flexibility.

Remember to focus on your breath and listen to your body throughout the Yoga Flow for Flexibility routine. If a pose feels uncomfortable or painful, modify it to suit your needs, or skip it altogether. The key is to move mindfully and with intention, allowing your body to relax and release tension with each breath.

Incorporating the Yoga Flow for Flexibility routine into your weekly workout schedule can profoundly impact your overall health and well-being. Spending just a few minutes each day practicing yoga can improve your flexibility, reduce stress, and enhance your physical performance in other activities. So, grab your mat, find a quiet space, and start flowing towards a more flexible and balanced body today.

Pilates for Posture and Balance

Pilates is a fantastic workout routine for improving posture and balance, making it a perfect addition to your home workout hustle. With its focus on core strength, flexibility, and alignment, Pilates can help you stand taller and move more gracefully throughout your day. Whether sitting at a desk for hours or running around after kids, Pilates can help counteract the effects of poor posture and muscle imbalances.

One of Pilates's key benefits is its emphasis on proper alignment and body awareness. By practicing Pilates regularly, you can train your body to maintain good posture even when you're not actively thinking about it. This can help alleviate common issues like back pain, neck stiffness, and shoulder tension, often caused by poor posture. Additionally, Pilates can improve your balance by challenging your stability and coordination in various exercises.

The good news is that incorporating Pilates into your busy schedule doesn't require a lot of time or fancy equipment. Many Pilates exercises can be done using just your body weight, making them perfect for a quick workout at home. Additionally, plenty of accessories, such as resistance bands, stability balls, and foam rollers, can enhance your Pilates practice. These tools can help deepen your stretches, increase your strength, and improve your balance.

To get started with Pilates for posture and balance, consider adding a few essential exercises to your daily routine. Moves like the Pilates Hundred, Roll-Up, and Swan Dive can target your core muscles and improve spinal alignment. Practicing these exercises regularly can strengthen your postural muscles, increase your flexibility, and enhance your overall balance. Remember to focus on proper form and alignment to benefit from each exercise the most.

In conclusion, Pilates is a great way to improve your posture and balance, even when you're short on time. By incorporating Pilates into your home workout routine, you can reap the benefits of better alignment, increased strength, and improved stability. Whether you're a beginner or a seasoned pro, Pilates offers a wide range of exercises that can help you achieve your health and fitness goals. So why not give Pilates a try and see the positive impact it can have on your posture and balance? https://www.verywellfit.com/pilates-posture-check-2704573

https://www.healthline.com/health/fitness/pilates-exercises

Chapter 5: Staying Consistent and Motivated

Setting Realistic Goals

Setting realistic goals is crucial when incorporating a home workout routine into your busy schedule. As a busy individual, it can be tempting to set lofty goals that may be difficult to achieve, given your time constraints. By setting realistic goals that are attainable within your current lifestyle, you can increase your chances of success and ensure that you stay motivated to continue your health journey.

Consider your current fitness level and schedule when setting goals for your home workout routine. It's essential, to be honest about how much time you can realistically dedicate to working out each week. If you only have 30 minutes to spare, setting a goal to exercise for two hours each day may not be practical. Instead, consider setting a goal to work out for 30 minutes five days a week. This way, you can easily incorporate your workouts into your daily routine without feeling overwhelmed.

Another important aspect of setting realistic goals is to make them specific and measurable. Instead of setting a vague goal like "I want to get in shape," try setting a more specific goal such as "I want to lose 10 pounds in the next three months." By making your goals specific, you can track your progress more effectively and make adjustments as needed. Additionally, setting measurable goals allows you to celebrate your achievements along the way, which can help keep you motivated.

In addition to setting realistic and specific goals, it's essential to make sure that your goals are achievable within your current circumstances. For example, if you don't have access to a treadmill or dumbbells, setting a goal that requires this specific equipment may not be feasible. Instead, focus on setting goals that can be achieved with your available resources. This will help you stay on track and avoid becoming discouraged if you encounter obstacles.

Setting realistic goals is critical to success when incorporating a home workout routine into your busy schedule. Consider your current fitness level, schedule, and available resources to set attainable and motivating goals. Remember to make your goals specific, measurable, and achievable, and don't be afraid to adjust them as needed. With the right mindset and approach, you can achieve your health and fitness goals while juggling a busy lifestyle.

Tracking progress and the many ways that they can track with mobile apps

Tracking progress is crucial to any fitness journey, especially for busy individuals who prioritize their health. With the rise of mobile apps, there are countless ways to track your progress and stay motivated. Whether using a fitness tracker, a calorie counting app, or a workout log, these tools can help you stay accountable and progress towards your health goals.

One popular way to track progress is through fitness tracker apps that monitor your steps, heart rate, and sleep patterns. These apps can provide valuable data on your daily activity levels and help you set realistic goals for improvement. With the ability to sync with other devices, such as smartwatches or fitness bands, you can easily track your progress throughout the day and stay on top of your fitness goals.

Calorie-counting apps are another valuable tool for busy individuals looking to improve their health. These apps can help you track your food intake, set calorie goals, and monitor your macronutrient intake. By recording your meals and snacks, you can gain valuable insights into your eating habits and make more informed choices about your nutrition. With features like barcode scanning and meal planning, these apps make it easy to stay on track, even when you're short on time.

For those who prefer structured workout routines, there are also apps available that can help you track your progress and stay motivated. These apps often include pre-designed workouts, exercise demonstrations, and progress-tracking tools to help you stay on track with your fitness goals. By logging your workouts and tracking your improvements over time, you can see your progress and stay motivated to keep pushing yourself.

In conclusion, tracking progress is essential for busy individuals looking to prioritize their health and fitness goals. With the convenience of mobile apps, there are countless ways to track your progress and stay motivated. Whether using a fitness tracker app, a calorie-counting app, or a workout log, these tools can help you stay accountable and progress toward your health goals. Utilizing these tools and staying consistent with your tracking can help you achieve your fitness goals and lead a healthier, more active lifestyle.

The immense Importance of Finding something or someone for accountability

Accountability is crucial to any successful health and fitness journey, especially for busy individuals who struggle to find time for regular exercise. Whether committing to a daily workout routine or a healthy eating plan, having someone or something to hold you accountable can make all the difference in achieving your health and fitness goals. This subchapter will explore the immense importance of finding something or someone for accountability in your home workout hustle.

One of the main benefits of having accountability in your fitness journey is the motivation it provides. Knowing that someone is counting on you to show up for a workout or stick to a healthy eating plan can be a powerful motivator to stay on track. This can be especially helpful for busy individuals who struggle to find the time or energy to exercise regularly. Having someone or something hold you accountable makes you more likely to stay committed to your health and fitness goals.

Another critical aspect of accountability is the sense of responsibility it instills in you. Knowing someone is watching or tracking your progress makes you more likely to take your health and fitness goals seriously. This can help you stay focused and disciplined, even when hectic. By having something or someone hold you accountable, you are more likely to make healthier choices and prioritize your well-being.

In addition to providing motivation and a sense of responsibility, accountability can help you track your progress and stay on course towards your goals. Whether using a fitness app to log your workouts, checking in with a workout buddy, or setting weekly goals, having accountability can help you stay organized and focused on your health and fitness journey. This can be especially useful for busy individuals who may struggle to remain consistent with their workouts or eating habits.

Overall, finding something or someone for accountability in your home workout hustle can be a game-changer for busy individuals looking to prioritize their health and fitness. Whether using accessories like dumbbells or a treadmill, partnering up with a workout buddy, or setting specific goals, accountability can help you stay motivated, responsible, and on track toward achieving your health and fitness goals. So don't underestimate the power of accountability in your home workout routine; it could be the key to unlocking your full potential and achieving the results you desire.

Celebrating small wins and the many ways that could look like for home workouts

Celebrating small wins is essential to staying motivated and committed to your home workout routine. It's easy to get discouraged when progress seems slow, but taking the time to acknowledge and celebrate the small victories along the way can make a big difference in your overall mindset and motivation. Whether completing an extra set of reps, reaching a new personal best, or simply showing up and putting in the effort, every small win is a step in the right direction.

Celebrating these small wins in your home workout routine can be done in many ways. One way is to treat yourself to a small reward, such as a healthy snack or a relaxing bath, after a particularly challenging workout. Another option is to track your progress and celebrate each milestone you reach, whether it's a new personal record or a certain number of workouts completed. Sharing achievements with friends or family can also be a great way to celebrate and stay accountable.

Incorporating accessories like dumbbells, treadmills, resistance bands, or yoga mats into your home workout routine can add a new dimension to your celebrations. For example, setting a goal to increase the weight you lift with your dumbbells or the speed you run on your treadmill can give you something concrete to work towards and celebrate when you achieve it. Using accessories like resistance bands or yoga mats can make your workouts more challenging and rewarding, giving you even more opportunities to celebrate your progress.

It's important to remember that celebrating small wins is not just about the end result but also about the journey and the effort you put in along the way. By focusing on the process and recognizing the hard work you're putting in each day, you can stay motivated and inspired to keep pushing yourself in your home workout routine. Remember, every small win is a step closer to reaching your goals and becoming the healthiest version of yourself.

In conclusion, celebrating small wins in your home workout routine is essential for staying motivated and committed to your health and fitness goals. Whether through rewards, tracking progress, or using accessories to challenge yourself, finding ways to celebrate your achievements can help you stay on track and continue making progress. So, take the time to acknowledge and celebrate your small wins, no matter how insignificant they may seem, and watch your motivation and commitment to your home workout hustle grow stronger each day.

Chapter 6: Tips for Busy Health Enthusiasts

Time Management Strategies

Time management is essential for busy individuals who want to prioritize their health and fitness goals. With the right strategies, even the busiest schedules can accommodate a home workout routine. One effective strategy is to schedule your workouts in advance and treat them as non-negotiable appointments. By setting aside dedicated time for exercise, you are more likely to stick to your routine and progress towards your fitness goals.

Another time management strategy for busy health enthusiasts is to make use of accessories that can enhance your home workout experience. Investing in equipment such as dumbbells, resistance bands, or a treadmill can help you maximize the effectiveness of your workouts in a shorter amount of time. These accessories can add variety to your routine and target different muscle groups, allowing you to make the most of your limited workout time.

Another critical time management strategy for busy individuals is prioritizing efficiency in workouts. High-intensity interval training (HIIT) workouts, for example, are a great way to maximize calorie burn and build strength quickly. By incorporating HIIT workouts into your routine, you can achieve significant results in as little as 20–30 minutes, making it easier to fit exercise into your busy schedule.

In addition to scheduling workouts, utilizing accessories, and prioritizing efficiency, time management for busy health enthusiasts also involves setting realistic goals and tracking progress. Establishing clear, achievable goals and tracking your workouts and progress can help you stay motivated and focused on your fitness journey. Whether you're aiming to increase your strength, improve your endurance, or lose weight, setting specific goals can help you stay on track and make the most of your home workout routine.

Effective time management is crucial for busy individuals who want to prioritize their health and fitness goals. By implementing strategies such as scheduling workouts, using accessories, prioritizing efficiency, and setting realistic goals, you can maximize your limited workout time and achieve the desired results. With the right mindset and commitment to your health, you can prioritize home workouts in your busy schedule and reap the benefits of a healthier, more vital, and more energized lifestyle.

Meal Planning and Prepping and different apps that can help with the process and tracking

Meal planning and preparation are essential components of maintaining a healthy lifestyle, especially for busy individuals who may not have the time to cook healthy meals every day. By planning and preparing meals in advance, you can ensure that you have nutritious options readily available, making it easier to stick to your health goals. Several apps are available that can help streamline the meal planning and preparation process, making it even easier for busy individuals to prioritize their health.

One popular app for meal planning and preparation is Mealtime. This app allows users to browse through a variety of healthy recipes and create personalized meal plans based on their dietary preferences. The app also generates a shopping list for each meal plan, making stocking up on the necessary ingredients easy. Another helpful app is Prepare, which helps users plan their meals and provides step-by-step instructions for preparing each dish. This can be especially helpful for individuals who may not be experienced in the kitchen.

In addition to meal planning and preparation apps, apps can help track your progress and keep you motivated on your health journey. MyFitnessPal is a popular app that allows users to track their daily food intake and exercise routines, helping them stay accountable and make healthier choices. Another app, Fitbod, provides personalized workout plans based on your fitness goals and preferences, making it easy to keep on track with your exercise routine.

By utilizing these apps, busy individuals can take the guesswork out of meal planning and preparation, making it easier to prioritize their health even when time is limited. Whether you're looking to improve your diet, track your progress, or find new workout routines, there are apps available to help you reach your health and fitness goals. Staying healthy and active can be more achievable with the right tools and resources.

Incorporating Workouts into a busy daily routine

Incorporating workouts into a busy daily routine can be challenging, but it is definitely possible with the right strategies and dedication. For busy individuals who want to prioritize their health and fitness, finding ways to squeeze in exercise can have numerous benefits for both physical and mental well-being. This subchapter will explore tips and tricks for incorporating workouts into a busy daily routine and the top 10 home workout routines that can help you stay on track with your fitness goals.

One of the first steps to incorporating workouts into a busy daily routine is to plan ahead. Look at your schedule for the week and identify pockets of time where you can fit in a quick workout. This could be early in the morning, before work, during your lunch break, or after dinner. By planning ahead and setting aside dedicated time for exercise, you are more likely to stick to your routine and make it a priority.

Another helpful tip for busy individuals looking to incorporate workouts into their daily routine is to use accessories that can make your workouts more efficient and effective. Investing in items such as dumbbells, resistance bands, a treadmill, or a yoga mat can help you create a convenient and accessible home workout space. These accessories can also add variety to your workouts and help you target different muscle groups for a well-rounded fitness routine.

When choosing the proper home workout routines, finding challenging and enjoyable exercises is essential. The top 10 home workout routines included in this book are designed to cater to a variety of fitness levels and preferences so you can find a routine that suits your needs and goals. Whether you prefer high-intensity interval training, strength training, or yoga, there is a workout routine for everyone in this book.

In addition to planning ahead, using accessories, and choosing the proper workout routines, staying motivated and consistent with your exercise regimen is essential. Set realistic goals for yourself, track your progress, and celebrate your achievements. Remember that consistency is critical when seeing results from your workouts, so make an effort to stick to your routine, even on the busiest days.

Incorporating workouts into a busy daily routine may seem daunting at first, but with the right strategies and mindset, it is definitely achievable. By planning ahead, using accessories, choosing the proper workout routines, and staying motivated and consistent, you can prioritize your health even when you have a packed schedule. This book's top 10 home workout routines are designed to help you stay on track with your fitness goals and make exercise a seamless part of your daily routine.

Chapter 7: Troubleshooting Common Challenges

Dealing with Interruptions: After a distraction, have something in place to get your mindset back on your workout, whatever that may look like for you.

Interruptions are bound to happen, especially when trying to squeeze in a workout at home amidst a busy schedule. It's essential to have a plan for when distractions arise so that you can quickly get back into the right mindset for your workout. After a distraction, take a moment to refocus and reset your intentions for the workout ahead. This could be as simple as taking a few deep breaths or doing a quick stretch to get your body ready for movement.

One helpful tool for getting back on track after an interruption is having a go-to playlist or motivational quote to help you regain your focus and energy. Music has the power to uplift and energize us, so having a playlist of your favorite workout tunes ready to go can help you quickly get back into the right mindset for your workout. Similarly, having a motivational quote or mantra that resonates with you can serve as a powerful reminder of why you're prioritizing your health and fitness in the first place.

Another helpful strategy for dealing with interruptions is to have a set routine or ritual before each workout. This could be as simple as lighting a scented candle, doing a few minutes of meditation, or even just putting on your workout clothes. By establishing a consistent pre-workout routine, you can signal to your brain that it's time to focus and get into workout mode, making it easier to bounce back from any distractions that may come your way.

In addition to mental strategies, having the right accessories on hand can help you quickly get back on track after an interruption. Whether it's a set of dumbbells, a resistance band, or a yoga mat, readily available equipment can make it easier to jump right back into your workout. Similarly, if you have a treadmill or stationary bike at home, consider keeping it in a dedicated workout space free from distractions so you can quickly resume your workout after any interruptions.

Overall, the key to dealing with interruptions during your home workout routine is having a plan to get back on track quickly. By establishing a pre-workout routine, having motivational tools on hand, and keeping the right accessories nearby, you can ensure that you're able to maintain your focus and momentum, no matter what distractions may come your way. Remember, prioritizing your health and fitness is worth the effort, so don't let interruptions derail your progress toward your goals.

Overcoming Plateaus and different ways to get motivated for a home workout, like music, podcasts, or audiobooks.

Plateaus are a common hurdle that many individuals face when trying to maintain a consistent home workout routine. It can be frustrating when you feel like you're no longer making progress or seeing results. However, it's important to remember that plateaus are a natural part of the fitness journey and can be overcome with the right strategies. One way to push through a plateau is to mix up your routine by trying different workouts or increasing the intensity of your current exercises. This can help shock your body into responding and prevent it from getting used to the same old routine.

Another effective way to overcome plateaus is to stay motivated and engaged in home workouts. One popular method is to listen to music while exercising. Music has been shown to enhance performance and increase motivation during workouts. Create a playlist of your favorite upbeat songs or high-energy tracks to keep you pumped and focused on your workout. You can also try incorporating motivational podcasts or audiobooks to keep your mind engaged and motivated while exercising.

In addition to music, incorporating accessories like dumbbells, resistance bands, or a treadmill can add variety and challenge to your home workouts. Dumbbells are versatile and can be used for a wide range of exercises to target different muscle groups. Resistance bands add resistance to body-weight exercises or target specific muscles. A treadmill can provide a convenient way to get a cardio workout without leaving home. Having these accessories on hand can make your workouts more enjoyable and effective.

Setting specific goals and tracking your progress can also help keep you motivated and focused on your home workouts. Whether you're aiming to increase your strength, improve your endurance, or reach a specific weight or body fat percentage, having clear goals can give you something to strive for. Keep track of your workouts, measurements, and progress photos to see how far you've come, and stay motivated to keep pushing forward.

Overall, overcoming plateaus and staying motivated for home workouts requires a combination of strategies. Mixing up your routine, listening to music, incorporating accessories, setting goals, and tracking your progress are all effective ways to keep yourself engaged and motivated. Remember that progress takes time and consistency, so don't get discouraged if you hit a plateau. Stay focused, stay positive, and keep hustling towards your health and fitness goals. https://www.healthline.com/nutrition/workout-plateau

Listening to your body is extremely important, but you can also push yourself a little bit harder to get the results you're looking for.

In the world of home workouts, listening to your body and understanding its limits is essential. However, pushing yourself a little harder can sometimes lead to better results. It's all about finding the balance between challenging yourself and avoiding injury. You can achieve your fitness goals more effectively by tuning into your body's signals and knowing when to push yourself.

When it comes to home workouts, having the right accessories can make a big difference in your results. Dumbbells, resistance bands, a treadmill, or even a yoga mat can all enhance your workout routine and help you push yourself to the next level. Investing in these accessories can make your workouts more effective and enjoyable, allowing you to see faster results.

If you're busy and want to prioritize your health, finding the time to exercise can be a challenge. That's why home workouts are a great solution—you can squeeze in a quick session whenever you have a free moment. By incorporating the right accessories and pushing yourself a little more, you can make the most of your limited time and see significant improvements in your health and fitness.

It's important to remember that progress takes time, and it's okay to start slowing and gradually increasing the intensity of your workouts. Pushing yourself too hard too soon can lead to burnout or injury, so listening to your body and making adjustments as needed is crucial. By gradually increasing the intensity of your workouts and paying attention to how your body responds, you can achieve sustainable results without compromising your health.

In summary, listening to your body is crucial when it comes to home workouts, but pushing yourself a little harder can help you achieve the results you're looking for. By investing in the right accessories and finding the right balance between pushing yourself and avoiding injury, you can make the most of your limited time and see significant improvements in your health and fitness. Remember to start slowing, gradually increase the intensity of your workouts, and always prioritize your health and well-being.

Chapter 8: Conclusion and Next Steps

Reflecting on Your Journey

As you near the end of your journey through the top 10 home workout routines in this book, it's essential to take a moment to reflect on how far you've come. You started this journey with the goal of making your health a priority, even with your busy schedule. You committed to carving out time each day to focus on your physical well-being, which is an accomplishment.

Reflecting on your journey can help you see how much progress you've made. Maybe you struggled to find the motivation to work out each day in the beginning, but now it's become a habit that you look forward to. Perhaps you started off with lighter weights or shorter cardio sessions, but now you find yourself pushing your limits and challenging yourself in new ways. By acknowledging and celebrating these small victories, you can stay motivated to continue your path to better health.

It's also important to take note of any obstacles you may have encountered along the way. Perhaps there were times when you felt discouraged by your slow progress or were too tired or busy to fit in a workout. Reflecting on these challenges can help you identify patterns or triggers that may derail your progress in the future. By recognizing these obstacles, you can come up with strategies to overcome them and stay on track toward your health goals.

As you reflect on your journey, consider the accessories instrumental in your success. Whether it's a set of dumbbells, a treadmill, resistance bands, or a yoga mat, these tools have helped you make the most of your home workouts. Take a moment to appreciate their convenience and versatility, allowing you to customize your routines and target different muscle groups. These accessories are not just tools; they affect your health and well-being.

In the final moments of your reflection, remember to pat yourself on the back for the dedication and effort you've put into your health journey. Making time for your well-being in the midst of a busy schedule is no easy feat, but you've shown that it's possible with commitment and perseverance. As you continue on your path to better health, carry this reflection with you as a reminder of how far you've come and how much you're capable of achieving. Your health is worth the hustle.

Setting New Goals and the importance of making a lot of small goals to get you to a larger goal

Setting new goals is essential in any fitness journey, especially for busy individuals who want to prioritize their health. It can be overwhelming to tackle a significant goal all at once, which is why breaking it down into smaller, achievable goals is vital. You can track your progress and stay motivated by setting small goals that align with your more substantial health and fitness objectives. This approach allows you to celebrate small victories and stay on track to reach your ultimate goal.

When it comes to home workouts, having a variety of goals is crucial. Whether you want to increase your strength, improve your cardiovascular fitness, or enhance your flexibility, setting specific goals for each area of fitness can help you stay focused and motivated. For example, if your ultimate goal is to run a 5k, setting smaller goals, such as increasing your running distance by 0.5 miles each week, can help you build up to your target distance over time. You can make steady progress toward your larger goal by setting achievable goals tailored to your fitness needs.

One of the benefits of setting small goals is that they are more manageable and less intimidating than tackling a big goal all at once. This approach allows you to focus on making incremental improvements each day rather than feeling overwhelmed by the enormity of your ultimate goal. You can build momentum and stay motivated throughout your fitness journey by breaking down your larger goal into smaller, more attainable steps. This strategy can help you stay on track and make consistent progress toward your health and fitness goals.

Incorporating dumbbells, treadmills, resistance bands, and other pieces of equipment into your home workout routine can help you achieve your fitness goals. These tools can add variety and challenge to your workouts, helping you build strength, improve endurance, and enhance flexibility. By setting specific goals for each accessory, you can tailor your workouts to target different muscle groups and achieve a well-rounded fitness routine. Whether you're looking to tone your arms with dumbbell exercises or increase your cardiovascular fitness with treadmill workouts, incorporating accessories into your routine can help you reach your fitness goals more effectively.

In conclusion, setting new goals and making many small ones to get you to a larger goal is essential for busy individuals who want to prioritize their health. By breaking down your larger fitness objectives into smaller, achievable goals, you can track your progress, stay motivated, and make steady improvements toward your ultimate goal. Incorporating dumbbells, treadmills, and resistance bands into your home workout routine can help you achieve your fitness goals more effectively. By setting specific goals for each area of fitness and incorporating accessories into your routine, you can create a well-rounded workout plan that aligns with your health and fitness objectives.

Continuing Your Home Workout Hustle apps that can help with that

In today's fast-paced world, finding the time to prioritize our health and fitness can be a challenge. However, with the right tools and resources, staying on track with your fitness goals is possible, even when you are short on time. One of the most convenient ways to stay active at home is by using workout apps that can help you stay motivated and focused on your goals. In this subchapter, we will explore some of the best workout apps that can help you continue your home workout hustle.

One of the top workout apps that can be a game-changer for busy individuals is the Nike Training Club app. This app offers a wide variety of workouts for all fitness levels, ranging from high-intensity interval training to yoga and strength training. With customizable workout plans and video tutorials, this app can help you stay on track with your fitness goals, no matter how busy your schedule.

Another excellent app for busy individuals is the MyFitnessPal app. This app can help you track your food intake and exercise routines to ensure that you are staying on track with your health and fitness goals. By inputting your meals and workouts into the app, you can stay accountable and make adjustments as needed to reach your desired results.

The Daily Burn app offers live and on-demand workout classes taught by licensed trainers for those who prefer a more guided approach to their home workouts. With a wide variety of workout styles, including cardio, strength training, and yoga, this app can help you stay motivated and engaged in your fitness routine.

If you are looking to track your progress and set new fitness goals, the Fitbod app can be a valuable tool. This app creates personalized workout plans based on your fitness level, goals, and equipment availability, making it easy to stay on track with your workouts and see tangible results over time.

In conclusion, incorporating workout apps into your home workout routine can be a game-changer for busy individuals who want to prioritize their health and fitness. Utilizing these apps allows you to stay motivated, track your progress, and keep on track with your fitness goals, no matter how busy your schedule. With the right tools and resources, you can continue your home workout hustle and achieve the results you desire.

www.ingramcontent.com/pod-product-compliance
Lightning Source LLC
Chambersburg PA
CBHW061027250726

48659CB00015B/2161